Healing from a Homebirth Cesarean

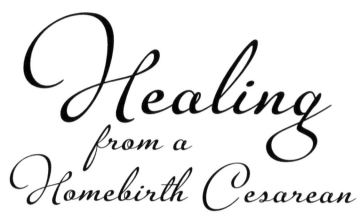

Healing
from a
Homebirth Cesarean

A companion workbook for any mother
whose planned out-of-hospital birth
ended in the operating room

Courtney Key Jarecki

Also by Courtney Key Jarecki

Homebirth Cesarean: Stories and Support for Families and Healthcare Providers

Printed in the United States of America
First Printing, 2015

ISBN 978-0-9862039-0-9

Incisio Press
Portland, Oregon
www.IncisioPress.com

For the daughters who gave everything to become mothers.

Success is about so much more than our vaginas.
And a cut in our bellies is not a failure.
—LEAH (2012/HBC, WESTERN U.S.)

And when it could do no more,
it learned, by God, it learned,
there may be endless
ways to open.
—WRITTEN BY SAGE, (2008/HBC, WESTERN U.S.)
FROM THE POEM *Dear Scar,*

Table of contents

·

Using this workbook

A homebirth cesarean (HBC) is the term used to describe a planned out-of-hospital birth that ended in the operating room. When women go from preparing and dreaming about a homebirth or birth center experience and relinquish those plans for a cesarean, the emotional fallout can be heavy.

As a compliment to the book, *Homebirth Cesarean: Stories and Support for Families and Healthcare Providers* (Incisio Press, 2015), this companion workbook provides mothers the space to continue their healing journey after their difficult or traumatic births. If you are seeking more information about the HBC experience, please refer to *Homebirth Cesarean: Stories and Support for Families and Health Care Providers.*

Before you begin please know that:

- This is your private journal. As you work through the exercises, do so with freedom knowing that what you write in here is for you alone.

- Release concerns about neatness, grammar, or staying in the margins. Use the entire workbook as your canvas. Spread out to larger pieces of paper when you want to.

- You may work through these exercises as slow or fast as you wish.

- Though the exercises are listed in a form that follows the HBC experience, complete them in any order that feels right to you.

- It is a good idea to identify a trusted support person who you can talk with if you become triggered or overwhelmed during an exercise.

- The information presented here is based on the work I've done in both writing the book *Homebirth Cesarean: Stories and Support for Families and Healthcare Providers* and facilitating workshops for birth professionals and healing retreats for mothers. Not every exercise will speak to your past or current experiences. These practices are meant to be applicable for many different women.

Useful tools

Because this can be emotionally challenging work, establishing a calming or grounding practice is beneficial and necessary. If you become upset during any of these exercises, try putting a hand on your heart as a way to calm your emotions and your mind. With your hand on your heart and your eyes closed, take a few deep, intentional breaths, returning to this work when you feel ready.

If you become overwhelmed during these exercises, please care for yourself. Maybe you need to take a break, put the workbook down, go outside, or make tea. Take deep breaths and decide if you want to tell a support person what is happening for you.

If you do not have a personal breathing or meditation practice, this simple exercise, originally offered in the book *Homebirth Cesarean,* may be supportive:

Close your eyes and feel your feet on the ground.
Observe your breath.
Take a deep inhale, then exhale.
Feel your breath entering
and exiting your lungs.
Do this several times.
Notice your emotions and thoughts.
Let them be.
Continue to breathe deeply, feeling your feet on the ground.
When you are ready, slowly open your eyes.

Chapter 1

Getting ready

Setting your intentions

Each mother has different reasons why she purchased this workbook. One woman's intention might be to heal from her birth trauma while another's simple wish may be to drive by the hospital without crying. So that you are clear on your intentions, list them below. Note that they may change as you work through these exercises.

Identifying triggers

Triggers are your nervous system's way of keeping you safe. If you fall through a sewer grate while walking down the street, your body will remember that experience every time you see sewer grates. Your heart rate and breathing will increase, you may begin to sweat, and you will feel scared even if you rationally know that the sewer grate you are approaching is not going to open.

As a mother who experienced a homebirth cesarean, you are here as a wounded warrior and a strong birthing woman. You may experience triggers at unsuspecting times, such as at the dentist, during routine pediatrician appointments, or as night approaches. So you can have greater awareness about what upsets you and returns you to a state of fear, anger, abandonment, grief, or trauma, list what has triggered you since your homebirth cesarean. Then write down all the ways you can imagine being triggered in the future. As you move through this workbook, come back to this list and add triggers you forgot or didn't even know existed.

For more information about triggers and the stress response during birth, refer to Chapter 3 in *Homebirth Cesarean: Stories and Support for Families and Health Care Providers.*

Past and current triggers

Possible future triggers

Your support network

Write the names of all the people you receive support from in your life. These people may be far away, only on the Internet, in your neighborhood, etc. Support can also come from online groups such as the "Homebirth Cesarean" Facebook group, or in-person women circles.

---------------------------------   ---------------------------------

---------------------------------   ---------------------------------

---------------------------------   ---------------------------------

---------------------------------   ---------------------------------

---------------------------------   ---------------------------------

---------------------------------   ---------------------------------

---------------------------------   ---------------------------------

------------------------------------   --

------------------------------------   --

------------------------------------   --

------------------------------------   --

------------------------------------   --

------------------------------------   --

Circle the names on your list of people you can call on to provide support. That support may be anything from walking the dog, holding your baby, listening to your birth story, or talking with you when you feel upset or triggered. Refer to this list when you need help or someone with whom to speak.

A special something

As homage to your strength as a woman, a birther, and a mother, find an object that is significant to you. It does not have to be birth or mother related. It can be anything you think is beautiful, sacred, or nice to hold; a rock, poem, picture, piece of art, etc.

Your object may not have any personal meaning to you now, but by the completion of this workbook it will represent your HBC healing path. This is your *special something*. This is yours that you can look at or hold to help ground you as you complete this workbook. It is your go-to when you feel triggered, upset, hopeless, sad, or happy.

Place your object where you have easy access to it.

My special something is:

Find that song

Music has the power to evoke emotions and shift moods. It also allows you to reach back in time and frame an experience. Choose a song to carry you through this workbook journey, something you want to hear when you are happy and sad. Listen to this song daily for the next 30 days.

My song for this journey is:

Chapter 2

The story you own

Your birth story now

Birth stories evolve as you heal and gain perspective on your experience. What begins as a highly upsetting and wounding story may hopefully become one of strength, relationship, and eventually power.

Write out your birth story. Take as long as you need to, using whatever medium you are drawn to, and start and stop as often as you wish. The more you write, the more details emerge—facts and perceptions you may have forgotten or dismissed come to light. Hurts that seemed embedded in your heart begin to vanish, answers to questions become clear, and your internal story begins to align with the story you tell others. Do not feel limited to the amount of space provided here—use extra paper as needed. In Chapter 5, you will be asked to re-write your birth story so you can compare the two versions.

Your ideal birth

On the lines provided list the components of your ideal, planned out-of-hospital birth. The spaces are short so you can focus on the key words of each intention. Examples might be: birth center, privacy, autonomy, loving, tenderness, connected, placenta medicine, etc.

From the list you just created, circle the components that were actually present during your HBC, even if they didn't take your ideal form. For example, though you did not have privacy in the hospital like you wanted, maybe you had a moment of privacy before the surgery. If that was the case for you, circle "privacy" as an element that was actually present during your homebirth cesarean.

Now, list some positive aspects from your HBC. Maybe you met new friends, learned about surgery recovery, found the perfect antidepressant, or discovered a strength in your partner or yourself you never knew existed. Over time, try to fill in all the lines and maybe even more.

---   ---

---   ---

---   ---

---   ---

What is most empowering

Identifying the most empowering moments during your HBC is a way to begin to heal your experience. Perhaps you loved that your partner held your hand during your entire labor at home, or you felt in-power when you were able to clearly listen to your midwife as she explained all your hospital induction options. Maybe the fact that you pushed at the birth center before transporting is an empowering time for you. As you begin to identify more of these moments, you may be able to let go of some of the disempowering ones and build a story that you can confidently share.

Identify at least five powerful moments during your birth.

1. ---

    ----

2. ---

    ----

3. --

----

4. --

----

5. --

Shifting your story

Motivation drives action. Shifting your birth story out of a place of hurt and into a place of strength, love, or power can be incredibly healing. List 3 reasons why shifting your birth story to one that better serves you is necessary:

1. --

----

2. --

----

3. --

Fairies and glue: Making changes

So many mothers worry that they will never find a birth story they feel comfortable telling their child. To help shake off the realities of your HBC, write a magical, fantasy version of your birth that includes a homebirth cesarean. Don't be limited by tangibility. Did fairies lift your baby out of your womb? Was your tummy sealed with an enchanted glue that makes it stronger than ever? Is your scar a secret symbol of strength that allows you access to your child? Use as many colorful, playful descriptions as you can. Have fun with this.

Pulling it together: A story for your child

Using the circled items from your ideal birth, the positive aspects from your HBC, your five powerful moments, and facets from your fairy tale birth, craft a story that you want to tell your child. Even if it feels inauthentic, or like you are forcing it, write it out. This is the beginning of an HBC story that you can be proud of—eventually growing to become the brave birth legend you will tell your child.

Checking in: Your support network

Have you used your support network listed in Chapter 1? Were you able to ask for help when you needed it? Write a few sentences about that.

How does it feel to accept and receive help?

Are there additional people you can think to add to your list of supporters? A social worker, a naturopathic doctor, your acupuncturist, a massage therapist, etc.? If so, write them here:

---   ---

---   ---

---   ---

---   ---

Combine this list and the list in Chapter 1 onto a separate piece of paper. This is a lineup of support, people to connect with when you need help or to talk. Hang it somewhere so you can see it everyday to remind yourself there are people in the world who want to help you, and that it is only a matter of you asking for help. If the help you are getting isn't the help you need, or if you can't find the right kind of assistance, keep asking. Keep searching. It is out there and you will find it.

Checking in: Triggers

Review your list of triggers in Chapter 1. Are there more you need to add?

Chapter 3

A time to be brave

Your birthing culture

All women carry into birth the spoken and unspoken beliefs of their families. Regardless of whether you subscribed to them or not, they still touched you in some way and helped shape your opinions of birth. Maybe your mother thought that other family members were weak for going to the doctor and that translated into you feeling shame for needing a cesarean. Perhaps your parents took you to the doctor for every little incident and you grew to resent that, which led to confusion and guilt about your birth. What messages did you receive as a child about birthing, hospitals, cesareans, and mothering? Take your time with this exploratory writing exercise. Think and feel into the ways your immediate family responded to situations around pain, pregnancy, birth, surgery, hospitals, trust, bodies, etc.

Pre-labor homebirth cesareans

Whether due to baby's position or health reasons, many women did not have a chance to experience labor out of the hospital or even feel contractions. These women had to transfer care to a hospital, perhaps use induction methods to begin labor, or move right into the operating room. If this is your story, write about how that aspect of your birth feels to you. Use full sentences or one word descriptions. Describe the unique feelings a pre-labor homebirth cesarean brings to your heart.

.

Making room inside

When you are able to identify specific hurts and move them out of your body and into an external place, you create space for profound healing. The following three steps walk you through this process.

1. Identify the hurts

Find a comfortable seated position. Feel your body on the ground, close your eyes, take a few deep breaths. Listen to your breathing.

Recall a conversation or interaction with your midwife, doula, lactation consultant, childbirth educator, doctor, or nurse that made you feel uneasy. Select one situation, and for the next few minutes, think about it as if you are observing it happening between two people you do not know. How does that situation feel? In your mind label the emotions with simple descriptions—scary, tense, upsetting, etc.

Quiet your mind. Take a few deep breaths, again feel your body on the ground. See those labels as thought bubbles. In your imagination, design and color them anyway you want. Maybe they are purple and green with rainbows spilling from some of the letters. Perhaps the labels look like graffiti with bright red ink dripping from the words. Anything goes.

As you see the words in your mind, acknowledge that those labels are how you feel about the interaction you had with your care provider. Speak the labels out loud. Just say the words. HURT. AFRAID. UNSUPPORTED. SO ANGRY.

Take ownership of those labels. Audibly say, "I feel hurt." or "I feel afraid." How do you feel after speaking them? Did it feel true? Did it feel awkward? Speak them again, this time powerfully, with conviction. "I FEEL HURT!" "I DO FEEL AFRAID!"

Take a few deep breaths. Feel your body on the ground. Open your eyes. Stretch your arms above your head. Stand up. Celebrate that which may have once been disconnected—an unsettling conversation or event—has now been identified, spoken out loud, and connected with who you are in this moment.

2. Get it out

Now that you've identified the emotions surrounding the event, you can begin to create the room to fully feel into it. Creating this space allows you to become less gripped by the event, less likely to get snagged by your emotions. By unlocking a hurt and putting it outside yourself, you can allow your intense emotions to become less charged and feelings may begin to soften.

Creating this room can take the form of journaling, drawing, performing a ritual, identifying an object that represents your hurt and burying it, burning it, or soaking it in salt water. Whatever feels good in the moment, you can do.

3. Repeat

Whenever you feel unsettled, bothered, or upset, set aside a few minutes to calm your mind and breath. Consider the upsetting incident, observe it as a witness, label the feelings, and take those labels outside of yourself into a physical object.

Checking in: Your calming and grounding practice

Have you been utilizing the meditation practice listed in the Introduction? Have you found something different that works for you? Spend a few minutes focusing on your breath, feeling your body on the earth, and quieting your mind.

Unenforceable rules

Each of us have personal rules that define how we act in situations and what we expect out of big events in our lives. Your out-of-hospital birth was an event where you probably had many hard and fast unenforceable rules—otherwise you wouldn't be working through these exercises. Examples of unenforceable rules are that homebirth is the safest way to birth, cesarean causes life-long problems, you deserved a happy postpartum experience, you should just be grateful to be a mother, etc. In the spaces below, identify the unenforceable rules you had for your birth, cesarean, the first few weeks postpartum, and motherhood prior to your HBC.

Out-of-hospital

1. --

2. --

3. --

4. --

5. --

Cesarean birth

1. --

2. --

3. --

4. --

5. --

Early postpartum

1. --

2. --

3. --

4. --

5. --

Motherhood

1. --

2. --

3. --

4. --

5. --

Now that you have crossed the homebirth cesarean threshold, you have been given the gift of experience that the unenforceable rules you set for yourself were not your reality. Write out how your unenforceable rules have changed in the wake of your HBC. Use a stream-of-conscious writing style: Do not lift your hand from the page, do not pause in your writing. Allow your thoughts to flow from your heart through your writing instrument and courageously wonder what you will write next.

Checking in: That special something

How has your *special something* been helpful to you so far? Describe how its meaning has changed, or if it has stayed the same. If you haven't been routinely connected to your object, write about why you think that is. Consider using a daily task, like eating an afternoon snack, as a reminder to connect with your *special something*.

Writing to see what comes

Using your non-dominant hand to write allows more access to unfiltered beliefs and stories you hold deep inside yourself. Find a marker, oil pastel, crayon, or other non-traditional writing instrument. You may need more pages than what is provided here, so have those at the ready. Set a timer for 15 minutes and take a moment to hold your writing tool in your non-dominant hand, feel your body connect to the earth, and then begin to write. Be unconcerned with what you are writing or the shape your letters take. Let your writing roam around between subjects as they arrive and/or occur to you. See what emerges. Write. Write. Right.

Forgiveness

After traumatic events there needs to be forgiveness before there can be healing. Forgiveness is a gift we give ourselves by letting go of anger, hurt, and resentment; it is a gateway to acceptance and healing. It does not absolve yourself or others from responsibility, but it does soften the grief you may feel. Who would you like to forgive? For what? Be detailed about the *whats* and include yourself in the *who*. Pull from all aspects of your experience—the natural birth community, your childbirth class, what you were taught as a youngster, etc.

Checking in: That song

Take a few minutes to listen to the song you choose at the start of this workbook. If you haven't been listening to it everyday, can you start that practice today and continue it for 30 days?

Your inner birth child

Your inner birth child is the part of you that so yearned for a peaceful experience for both you and your baby. It's the part of you that feels hurt, betrayed, and maybe unloved. It's the part of you that requires compassion, nurturing, and tenderness to heal.

To get in tune with your inner birth child, write simple words and sentences that a child might use to describe the hurt you feel as a result of your HBC. *I'm angry!!!!!, I hate everything, ARRRGGGGGGHHH!!!* are examples of what might be going on for an inner birth child. Make your words as large and colorful as a child might.

.

Maintaining that same mindset, write out what your inner birth child needs from you, the adult, to help heal her wounds. You might find yourself writing things like love, help, hungry for cookies. Keep the words and sentences simple, and read with childlike fascination what your inner birth child has to say.

Placenta medicine

Perhaps you are one of the many women who lost their chance to bury, make medicine, hold ceremony, or even see their placentas after surgery. If you yearn to close the circle with the organ that nourished your baby, holding a placenta burial, even if you aren't actually in possession of your placenta, can be very healing.

If you no longer have your placenta, find something that represents it. This can be a piece of fruit, a rock, fabric, flowers, anything at all. How you choose to design your placenta burial ceremony is up to you. You can wrap your object in fabric, put it in a shoebox, or bury it directly in the ground. Perhaps you want loved ones with you or you choose to perform this ceremony solo. Maybe you light a candle or a larger fire as you dig a hole to bury your placenta. There could be a festive drink or meal afterwards or quiet time away from your baby.

After the placental ceremony, go to your *special something* you selected at the start of this workbook. Spend a few minutes with it. Sit with it. Let it take on any difficult feelings you may not be ready to deal with at this time.

Chapter 4

Your scar, your body

Self-massage

As a way to re-integrate your body, begin a practice of self-massage for three minutes everyday. This practice can help your body feel whole and complete again.

On day-one, start by massaging your feet. Make this an intentional practice, something that begins and ends with a few deep breaths, your only focus is on your hands rubbing that specific body part. Each day pick a new body part to massage, with the goal of eventually, when you are ready, massaging your scar. Do this practice daily for 30 days and set a calendar reminder to help you integrate it into your life.

Belly mandalas

Mandala, loosely translated from Sanskirt, means circle. Mandala circle art traditionally represents wholeness, and can be used as a modern day practice to help focus attention. In this exercise you will be creating three mandalas, each one representing different parts of your HBC journey. Use any mediums you wish: pastels, markers, crayon, pencil, paint, collage, etc. Before you begin each mandala, take a moment to ground yourself and connect with your center.

The first mandala: Create a picture of your belly before your cesarean. Recall a pregnancy memory. Invoke the feelings from that memory to begin drawing your pre-HBC belly.

The second mandala: Draw a picture of your belly after your cesarean. This may be a triggering or overwhelming exercise, so go slow and use the grounding and breathing practices you have developed throughout this workbook. Remember that this isn't the last mandala you are asked to draw, so you won't get emotionally stuck here with just these two pictures.

Take a moment to ground yourself and connect with your center. Recall a memory from your birth—positive or negative. Invoke the feelings from that memory to begin drawing your cesarean belly.

Before continuing with the mandala drawing, take a moment to center yourself. In the book *Homebirth Cesarean*, Tami Lynn Kent, a woman's health physical therapist, shared the following meditation to help restore the energy between mother and child and bring the mother a beginning sense of peace. A more complete description of this meditation is in Kent's book, *Mothering from Your Center*. Read her meditation here, find a comfortable position with one hand on your heart and the other hand on your scar, then guide yourself through this meditation.

Picture your child the age they are now and then picture them as a newborn on your chest. Breathe that birth energy down your womb, through your cesarean incision, and up to your chest, making an imprint from womb to heart. Then let the energy go to your child at the age they are now and allow it to fill up their energy field. Allowing the birth energy to flow through your scar honors their birth process and brings healing as well.

Reflect on how you feel after the scar meditation:

The third mandala: Holding onto that same feeling from after Tami Kent's meditation, while keeping in mind that your incision is the birth site of your child, draw your belly now.

Reflect on how you feel after the completion of your three mandala pieces:

Checking in: Your song

Consider how listening to the song you identified earlier in the workbook has supported you through this journey? Does it still seem appropriate? If not, search for a new song. Do you listen to it when you drive? At home or work? Privately with headphones? Discover all the ways you can integrate this music into your life.

Nourishing bath

As a mother it can be difficult for you to take time for yourself. Despite the many directions you are pulled, spending 10 minutes in hot water can reenergize and invigorate your spirit in a way that is unique and healing. Find someone to tend to household needs while you are bathing. If you have a bathtub, light a few candles and pour epsom salt (or any salt you have handy) into the running water. Salt has the ability to relax the nervous system and ease tired muscles. If you have a favorite essential oil, add a few drops to the water. If you don't have a bathtub, take a long, hot shower and rub the salt on your body, along with any essential oil. Take your time leaving the bathroom, even if your family wants your attention. Soak in the steam and heat, close your eyes, and breathe deeply. If possible, immediately crawl into bed and rest. Try to do this once a week for 30 days, setting a calendar reminder can help create this into a routine.

Oh, that scar

The next few exercises focus on your scar. If this feels overwhelming, as it does for many mothers, come back to this section another time. And please remember your grounding and meditation exercises when you decide to begin.

Describe the first time you saw your scar.

Reflect on the most recent time you saw your scar.

List words to describe what it is like for you to touch your scar. Maybe it feels empowering, sad, icky, disconnected, loving, powerful, etc. All those descriptions can be true at the same time.

--   --

--   --

--   --

--   --

--   --

--   --

--   --

--   --

Scar exploration

For most mothers touching their scars is not easy. However, not doing so is a loss of connection to both a sacred birth site as well as your body. Even if touching your scar feels like the last thing you ever want to do, consider trying it. You can stop at any time. You are in control. Be gentle with yourself. Take breaks when you need to. Breathe. Allow yourself to fully experience this exploration, but don't push yourself too far too soon.

Set a timer for five minutes. Find a comfortable, reclining position. Relax into your breathing. Remove all clothing from your scar, place your hands on your chest, then slowly, with awareness of your breathing, move your hands towards your scar.

Write a description of your scar through your fingertips:

Try to touch your scar daily for 30 days. Even if touching means a purpose-
ful brush of the fingertips while dressing, that is a great start. To help tune
into your experience, you can select prompts from the list provided and
then begin to come up with your own. Focusing on a different prompt of
observation each time will help attune your attention and make it a little
easier to begin exploring.

Reflect on your perceptions after each session using the blank pages in the
back of this book for your notes.

Scar prompts

- What colors do you picture when you touch your scar?

- Feel your scar as if your child were touching it. How might your child
  describe the site of his or her birth?

- Notice sensations that come up in other parts of your body when
  touching your scar. What do you make of those sensations?

- To help re-imagine your scar, what animal does your scar remind
  you of?

- If your scar could talk, what would it say?

- If your scar was a Hollywood actress, what is her favorite movie genre?

- If your scar had a ringtone, what would it sound like?

- If a unicorn had a cesarean scar, how would she touch it?

- Your personal scar prompts listed here:

The scar plan

What are all the healing modalities (essential oils, acupuncture, massage, etc.) that you want to try to help your scar heal? Use the blank pages in the back of this book as a reminder in the months and years to come to pursue this healing.

Intimacy and sex

For many women, the scar from their surgical birth may make intimacy and sex more difficult. Mothers, regardless of how they gave birth, have a different sex life than they did before their baby—hormones have changed along with schedules, responsibilities, and free time. How has your intimacy and sex life changed since your HBC?

Of the ways your intimacy and sex life has changed, which do you attribute to your HBC and why?

Imagine that for a 24-hour period you and your partner had no baby to take care for, no responsibilities, and all the privacy a secluded and romantic vacation spot could offer. How would the two of you spend your time together? What would you do (sexual or not)? What would you talk about? What foods would you eat?

Combining your fantasy 24-hour vacation with your real life, what aspects of intimacy and sexuality can you actually bring into your current reality? How can you go about doing that?

Checking in: Self-massage reflection

Remember that self-massage practice for 30 days at the beginning of this chapter? How has that intentional practice of massage changed your relationship with your body? If you haven't been practicing self-massage, explore why that might be.

Chapter 5

Healing

State a declaration

A declaration is a pronouncement or assertion about the present or the future. It is something that can be true today or something you intend to be true in the future. A declaration can be anything: I want to heal. I want to love my scar. I want to sleep well tonight. I want to be more at ease. List 5 declarations you have in the present moment.

1. ....

2. ....

3. ....

4. ....

5. ....

To step into your declarations more deeply, re-write your declarations in the present tense. Your statements might read: I am healing. I sleep well. I am at ease. Before doing this, take a few deep, centering breaths to feel into your declarations.

1. ....

2. ....

3. ....

4. ---

5. ---

Using the present tense version of your declarations, stand up, feel your feet on the ground, and say them out loud. Maybe even do this in front of a mirror so you can see the power in your body as you speak.

How do you feel after speaking your declarations?

When speaking your declarations out loud, where in your body do you feel the most energy? The most power? What insights did you gain?

As part of an ongoing practice, speak your declaration everyday for the next 30 days. To help remember this, connect the declaration with a daily activity. Maybe you speak your declaration as you put toothpaste on your toothbrush, or while you are going to the bathroom, etc.

Checking in: Scar exploration

Have you been spending a few minutes every day tenderly touching your scar? If this is difficult for you, reflect on why that might be.

Thank yourself

As women and mothers it can be difficult to appreciate and thank ourselves. Spend 10 minutes writing a thank you card to yourself. Find a card that resonates with you, then write. Your gratitude can be about anything—how you birthed, how you nourish your baby, what a great mother you are, etc. Try to touch on all aspects of your life including partnerships, friendships, your life as a neighbor, worker, carpool driver. Keep your card in a visible place where you have easy access to it and can read it when you need to remind yourself about the wonderful work you do.

Checking in: Your special something

That object that you've had with you during this journey—the one that symbolizes your love and heartbreak, your scar and strength. The one you would bring to a gathering of other HBC mothers and hold in your hands as you listened to their stories. Look deeply at it now. Hold it. What is it saying it you?

Your birth story now

You began this workbook by writing your birth story. Now it is time to write it once again. As you settle into this exercise, you may notice new places of feeling in-power during your birth. Perhaps some of the hurts have become diminished. Welcome the new aspects of your story and keep writing until it is all out on paper.

.

Chapter 6

Another baby,
another birth

This chapter is for mothers who want to explore the possibility of having another child and/or are already pregnant. Healing from a homebirth cesarean does not happen with a subsequent vaginal birth, the healing begins before another pregnancy and is deepened between births.

There is a myth that having a VBAC (vaginal birth after cesarean) makes you a stronger birther, a warrior, or more of a woman. While you are likely to feel ecstatic and validated if you are able to push a baby out your vagina, what happens if you can't? What if you have another cesarean? What if the VBAC is more traumatic than your HBC? What if another birth reignites pain from your HBC? These exercises help you discover answers to these questions while supporting all birthing plans, including scheduled cesareans.

The decision process: Another birth
If you had to make a decision on where and how you would give birth today, what would that decision be? Would you birth at home? A birth center? In the hospital? In the operating room? Write out your current thinking that got you to this conclusion.

.

The next four exercises center on teasing apart the decision process around having another baby. Many HBC mothers worry that the may have a "hidden agenda" about wanting to become pregnant again so they can try for a successful VBAC. These listing exercises will help unpack your desires and intentions. As you brainstorm the answers, don't judge what you write. Let it all out. Doing this allows you to look at it from all angles, discard what you don't want, and strengthen what you wish.

What do you want from the next birth experience? List all your reasons in as few words as possible. For example, instead of writing that you want to feel the power of pushing a baby out your vagina, shorten your answer to *power*. Maybe on the next line write *pushing*. Keeping your answers in short form will allow you to see the key word(s) behind each intention. Use this format for the next four exercises.

--   --

--   --

--   --

--   --

--   --

Why do you want another baby?

--   --

--   --

--   --

--   --

--   --

--   --

--   --

--   --

--   --

--   --

-----------------------------------   -----------------------------------

-----------------------------------   -----------------------------------

-----------------------------------   -----------------------------------

-----------------------------------   -----------------------------------

-----------------------------------   -----------------------------------

What fears do you have about giving birth again?

-----------------------------------   -----------------------------------

-----------------------------------   -----------------------------------

-----------------------------------   -----------------------------------

-----------------------------------   -----------------------------------

-----------------------------------   -----------------------------------

-----------------------------------   -----------------------------------

-----------------------------------   -----------------------------------

-----------------------------------   -----------------------------------

-----------------------------------   -----------------------------------

-----------------------------------   -----------------------------------

--- ---

--- ---

--- ---

--- ---

--- ---

What fears do you have about the postpartum time?

--- ---

--- ---

--- ---

--- ---

--- ---

--- ---

--- ---

--- ---

--- ---

--- ---

--- ---

---   ---

---   ---

---   ---

---   ---

---   ---

Checking in: Nourishing bath

Can you take a bath tonight? What about tomorrow? If you are unable to plan for a nourishing bath, what is standing in your way?

The conversation now

If you are partnered, how does your partner feel about having another baby? What concerns does he or she have about childbirth? If you haven't had conversations about this, write out how you imagine he or she feels and what they would say. As you write, give yourself permission to add your own thoughts and feelings.

The support you might need

List the ways you believe you will need support from a partner or other trusted person during pregnancy, labor, birth, and postpartum. Write the names of people who you believe will be best at offering that support. For example, in the postpartum time you think you will need help breastfeeding and the people who can help you could be your partner, a lactation consultant, your step-mother, etc.

I need the following support during pregnancy:

I need the following support during labor and birth:

I need the following support during the postpartum:

Childbirth options: Take off your reality hat

You may not want to plan a homebirth, or another cesarean, but in these writing exercises you are asked to take off your reality hat and pretend, with all your heart and the gusto of a child, that you do want each of the options presented.

This section may fatigue and drain you, so pace yourself, go slow, and do try to complete it, even if it takes weeks or months. The intention is to help clear the clutter around what may happen in your next birth and give you room to see what you might want, and maybe even choose to have a different type of birth than you can imagine for yourself right now. So, pretend away.

Write about why you are planning an out-of-hospital birth. Detail your plans. Let your words flow as you describe how having a birth like this might make you feel. When writing about why you want a homebirth or birth center birth, do so with enthusiasm and and tenderness as if this is your first choice.

This time plan a hospital VBAC. Describe your ideal hospital birth and why you are looking forward to birthing in the hospital. Plan the support you will receive in the hospital, the compassionate conversations with staff, your choice-points at each intervention, etc. If this is the furthest from your actual heart's desire, be silly and have fun with it. Write about how you can't wait to have bright lights shining on your vagina and a crowd of people admiring your pushing skills. Be playful.

Here, write about the awesome cesarean birth you are planning. This is your birth, the one you want, so narrate how the scene unfolds, how the doctors and staff introduce themselves to you and your baby, how your arms are untied, how the spinal epidural makes you feel calm and relaxed. Paint the scene with words (or images) and, if you need to, pretend you are someone else writing this, someone who truly wants this for herself and her child.

Plan C: The cesarean birth plan

Regardless of the birth plans you make, you may feel called to create a Plan C. Even if you don't want a cesarean, keep in mind that not thinking about cesarean won't make your chances of having one go away. Plan C will only serve to educate and empower you if you are heading for the operating room.

If a scheduled cesarean is your first choice in birthing options, or the only one you are left with because of physical or mental health issues, Plan C will walk you through some of the options that may be available to you in the operating room. However, just with any hospital birth plan, it is unlikely that you will have access to all your wishes. By exploring the many options provided here, a family, together with their birth team, can identify one or two key needs in the event of an HBC and advocate for those items before consenting to a cesarean.

Directions for use:

1. Beginning with the "Before the cesarean" section, circle the bulleted option(s) you would like to have during a surgical birth. Feel free to add any additional items.

2. Review the items you have circled and, from those points, identify one or two non-negotiables. Write those in the Summary section. The Summary section allows your birth team to quickly note what is most important to you in the event of a cesarean.

3. Considering what you have circled and what is in your heart when you think about your ideal birth, list what your key needs and highest intentions are for a surgical birth. For example, your key needs may be that you are able to hold your baby in the OR and your highest intention might be that your body is treated with respect and at the baby's sex is not announced.

Summary

Non-negotiable options before consenting to a cesarean:

Key needs for a cesarean:

Highest intention for a surgical birth:

Before the cesarean

- I would like a few minutes alone with my partner before consenting / leaving for the operating room.

- I want to meet and speak with the OB who will be performing my surgery.

- I request both my partner and midwife/doula to provide support in the OR.

- If I do not have an epidural, I would like to walk to the OR.

- I do not want medical residents in the OR during my birth.

- If I require IV antibiotics, I want them to be given post-cord clamping so my baby does not receive the antibiotics.

In the OR—Mother

- I request that all staff in the OR introduce themselves and say hello to my baby.

- I would like a moment of silence in the OR before the surgery begins.

- I understand that trembling is normal and I do not want to be given anti-shaking medications.

- Do not tie my arms down.

- Keep casual conversation outside the OR.

- I want my support person to take photos in the OR.

- I would like a mirror so I can watch the birth of my baby.

- I would like the screen lowered as my baby is being born.

- I want to keep my placenta. If you need to send my placenta to the lab, take a small sample and leave the rest for me. Do not put my placenta in any preservatives.

- I prefer suturing over staples and request a clear bandage like Suture Strip Plus over my entire incision rather than Steri-Strips. I understand that using sutures may shorten my healing time and possibly result in a more cosmetically appealing scar.

In the OR—Baby

- Do not announce the sex.

- I request immediate skin-to-skin contact.

- Do not bathe, clean, swaddle, or footprint my baby.

- I want to begin breastfeeding in the OR.

- I request delayed cord cutting.

- I want my partner to cut the baby's cord after it is done pulsing.

Reminders for the partner in the OR and after the birth

- Pull down your mask, smile, kiss me, tell me I am strong.

- Only wear a scrubs overcoat, not a shirt, so our baby can be skin-to-skin with you.

- Tell me what is happening during the surgery / remain quiet during the birth unless I ask a question.

- Stay with the baby. Keep your hand on the baby. Talk to the baby. Insist on holding our baby.

- Do not introduce our baby to family or friends. I want that privilege.

- If our baby is in the NICU, do not show me pictures. Do not share pictures with anyone. If our baby is in the NICU, take a lot of pictures and videos.

- Do not text or email photos or post about the birth on social media without checking with me first.

Postpartum support network in the hospital

Call _____ to take care of the children at home.

Call _____ to take care of our pets.

Call _____ to bring what we need from home.

Call _____ to start our meal train at the hospital / when we get home.

Call _____ to clean our home before we are discharged.

Postpartum support network at home

Call _____ to meet us at home when we are discharged.

Call _____ to stay with me during the day.

Call _____ to stay with me during the night.

Call _____ to help with childcare of older siblings.

Call _____ to help with our pets.

Call _____ to pick up groceries and supplies.

Call _____ to help with household chores.

Call _____ to keep me company.

Closing

Mama, you are amazing. You surrendered to the pain of the scalpel so you could hold your baby. You walked through the fire of homebirth cesarean and you came out stronger. You had the courage to search deep in yourself for the answers and you decided to heal. You worked through these exercises and you have more understanding. You did this for yourself, your baby, and your family. Your strength is palatable.

What did you learn from completing these exercises?

.

LIST OF EXERCISES

BIOGRAPHY

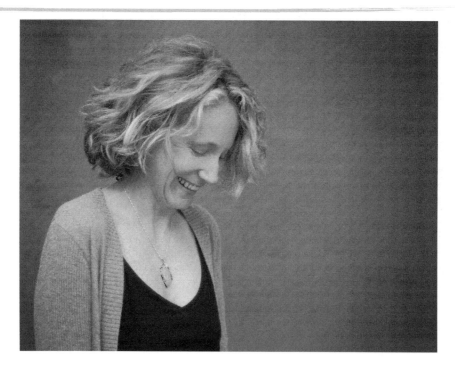

Courtney Key Jarecki has worked as a doula, childbirth educator, and a homebirth midwifery apprentice, but her path forever shifted after the birth of her daughter. In recovering from her 54-hour home labor, hospital transport, and cesarean, Courtney soon began creating a new model of understanding for these types of births, now known as *home-birth cesareans (HBC)*, a term she coined. Left without stories that reflected her own journey, she was driven to provide others with resources and support she could not find for herself.

Courtney envisions a future where women of her daughter's generation will birth with knowledge and dignity regardless of location, and in the company of care providers who respect and understand their wishes. She is the founder of the Homebirth Cesarean movement and is actively working to broaden the conversation and education around homebirth cesareans through the support of mothers, families, and birth professionals.

She envisions a future where women of her daughter's generation will birth with knowledge and dignity regardless of location, and in the company of care providers who respect and understand their wishes.

To attend an in-person or online workshop for birth professionals or a healing retreat for mothers who experienced an HBC, visit www.CourtneyJarecki.com

In balancing her writing, teaching, and leadership activities, she is also a mama to Lazadae, wife to Dave, and alpha-female pack leader to hounds Satchel and Maji. She lives in Oregon.

Made in the USA
Columbia, SC
05 August 2021